The answer to my prayer: Date:_______________

Today's Prayer: Date:_______________

____

____

____

____

____

____

____

____

____

____

____

____

____

____

____

____

____

____

____

____

____

When Jesus' disciples asked him why they couldn't drive out the demon from the man; *"He replied, "This kind can come out only by prayer."* (Mark 9:28-30) NIV

With the turmoil happening in our world or in our lives, there's only one way that we can combat that…through prayer.

For the next 30 days challenge yourself to not only pray but see how God responds to your prayers.

- ❖ Pray for someone or something daily

- ❖ Write down your prayers on each page

- ❖ See how God responds to your specific prayer – write that down on the opposite page – it may not be on the same day, so make sure to date them

- ❖ As each prayer is answered – either fold or tear off a corner of the page

- ❖ In the end, you'll see just how much God has been listening to you.

Today's Prayer: Date:_______________

The answer to my prayer: Date:_______________

Today's Prayer: Date:_______________

The answer to my prayer: Date:____________

Today's Prayer: Date:_______________

The answer to my prayer: Date:_____________

Today's Prayer: Date:_______________

The answer to my prayer: Date:_______________

Today's Prayer: Date:_______________

The answer to my prayer: Date:_____________

Today's Prayer: Date:_____________

The answer to my prayer: Date:_______________

Today's Prayer: Date:_______________

The answer to my prayer: Date:_______________

Today's Prayer: Date:_______________

____

____

____

____

____

____

____

____

____

____

____

____

____

____

____

____

____

____

____

The answer to my prayer: Date:_____________

Today's Prayer: Date:_______________

The answer to my prayer: Date:_______________

Today's Prayer: Date:_______________

The answer to my prayer: Date:______________

Today's Prayer: Date:_______________

The answer to my prayer: Date:____________

Today's Prayer: Date:_______________

The answer to my prayer: Date:_____________

Today's Prayer: Date:______________

The answer to my prayer: Date:_______________

Today's Prayer: Date:_______________

The answer to my prayer: Date:_______________

You may write down all the answered prayers here
for a quick glance.
*"Therefore I tell you, whatever you ask for
in prayer, believe that you have received it, and it
will be yours."* (Mark 11:24)

Date: _______________________________

Date: _______________________________

Date: _______________________________

Date: _______________________________

Date: _______________________________

Date: _______________________________

Date: _______________________________

Date: _______________________________

Date: _______________________________

Date: _______________________________

Date: _______________________________

Date: _______________________________

Date: _______________________________

Date: _______________________________

Date: _______________________________

Date: _______________________________

Date: _______________________________

Date: _______________________________

Date: _______________________________

Date:

Date:

Date:

Date:

Date:

Date:

Date:

Date:

Date:

Date:

Date:

Date:

Date:

Date:

Date:

Date:

Date:

Date:

Date:

Date:

Date:

Date:

Date:

Date: